Paleo Diet Blueprint

Beginners Guide for Weight Loss

Copyright © 2015 by Bora Gyeong

Disclaimer

This book is designed to provide information on the Paleo diet only. This information is provided and sold with the knowledge that the publisher and author do not offer any legal or other professional advice. In the case of a need for any such expertise consult with the appropriate professional. This book does not contain all information available on the subject. This book has not been created to be specific to any individual's or organizations' situation or needs. Every effort has been made to make this book as accurate as possible. However, there may be typographical and or content errors. Therefore, this book should serve only as a general guide and not as the ultimate source of subject information. This book contains information that might be dated and is intended only to educate and entertain. The author and publisher shall have no liability or responsibility to any person or entity regarding any loss or damage incurred, or alleged to have been incurred, directly or indirectly, by the information contained in this book. You hereby agree to be bound by this disclaimer or you may return this book within the guarantee time period for a full refund.

Table of Contents

Introduction

The Paleo diet dates back to man's ancestors. Going back to the root of mankind, men hunted with their bare hands, fished, and lived off the land by eating what could be found in the wild. Packed with protein, the Paleo diet can be every man's dream come true. Tackling the Paleo diet can mean ignoring many of the foods that are widely advertised in today's society. The Paleo diet means looking to the cavemen for answers on both health and nutrition. When your goal is overall health, you need to consider two main factors: diet and exercise. Diets aren't just used for men who want to lose weight but also for general overall health. Benefits to a healthier lifestyle through the Paleo diet can be endless and unmeasurable for many.

Chapter One: Current Health Problems

There is no argument that the average person's diet has changed drastically over the years. There is double the amount of fast-food restaurants today compared to 1970. Today's average American consumes above the recommended intake of calories, grains, sodium, and saturated fat while continuing to decrease the amount of recommended servings of fruits and vegetables. Statistics show that 25% to 40% of Americans are obese. Why is this such a problem? A recent study showed that 52% of Americans believed that doing their taxes was easier than figuring out how to eat healthy. Over one out of every four people eat some type of fast food every day. The problems that many Americans are facing today are time constraints and lack of knowledge in how to eat correctly. Agricultural advancements and preservative use may be a cause of increased obesity in the United States. Popular diets that include highly processed food coupled with lack of exercise may also be the cause of increased disease processes. Evidence has shown that over time, our bodies adapt and evolve to our culture, but our systems may not have been ready for the hasty change of food and lifestyle. There is an increase of diet-related diseases such as obesity, cardiovascular disease, and diabetes. One in every four American deaths is related to cardiovascular disease. Heart disease increases the chance of other conditions such as diabetes, stroke, obesity, physical inactivity, and mental illness. These diseases are not only increasing in frequency but also their onset is evident in younger age groups. Children below the age of sixteen are dealing with disease processes normally seen in age groups above forty. Many disease processes aren't natural in the body system. People aren't born with most of the plaguing diseases we see today. The diseases seen today were created by the eating and lifestyle choices of people.

Chapter Two: Health Benefits

The Paleo diet consists of what our bodies have been using for thousands of years. Coupled with exercise, the Paleo diet can aid in heart health, diabetes prevention, and lowering cholesterol. The high lean-protein dietary focus can create more efficient workouts with greater results. The fruits-and-vegetables focus can assist in stabilizing blood sugars, burning stored fat, reducing allergies, increasing and balancing energy, clearing skin, and improving sleep patterns. Using the Paleo diet with the goal of overall health will move the body into a natural state, giving the body what it needs through a decrease in blood sugar, blood pressure, and cholesterol, weight loss, control of stomach problems, and increased mental health and self-esteem. The Paleo diet is a clean and healthy living lifestyle.

Chapter Three: Paleolithic Era

The Paleo diet refers to the Paleolithic age of man. The word "Paleo" refers to a Greek term meaning "old," and "lithic" originates from a Greek word meaning "stone." The word Paleolithic can be translated to "the Stone Age." The Paleolithic era comprises approximately 90% of man's life on earth. It was a primitive time marked by stone tools that spanned from 2.6 million years ago to approximately 10,000 years ago. The earliest human fossils were dated to over one million years ago, located in Kenya, Tanzania, and Ethiopia. The Paleolithic era can also be described as the "hunter-gatherer" time period that spanned through the Ice Age. Men hunted wild animals for meat and gathered food, firewood, and materials for tools, clothes, and shelter. Humans formed groups of small societies and thrived by gathering plants, fishing, hunting, and scavenging off the land for wild animals. Early humans lived in forests, which allowed them to survive on fish, eggs, nuts, fruits, and vegetables. It was found that Paleolithic humans would scavenge for meat from already-deceased animals found in the wilderness rather than hunting themselves. This was thought to be because of the dangers associated with hunting large game in that era. Mammals such as woolly mammoths, woolly rhinoceros, and cave lions inhabited the earth during this time.

During the Paleolithic era, the climate consisted of fluctuating warm and ice-cold glacial temperatures. The time period is known to have had weather changes that forced the movement of colonies to warmer areas where food, such as plants and animals, were readily available. It is theorized that the drifting of continents took place during this time period, as many artifacts originating in southern Africa were found Asia, Europe, and the Americas. This is supported by the idea that humans were unable to cross large bodies of water with the available technology. As Africa drifted further south, the cold

Antarctic Ocean made it difficult for survival. Along with ice sheets, the cold, dry air forced early humans to migrate further north. The Paleolithic era is known to have finished through the end of the ice age, when the earth's climate became warmer. A majority of our knowledge of Paleolithic lifestyles and nutritional intake comes from archeology, theories, and comparisons to modern day hunter-gatherer societies.

Chapter Four: Agriculture

Agriculture is the cultivation of land for animals, plants, life forms for food, fuel, medicine, and products that enhance human life. Researchers believe that our metabolisms have not been able to adapt quickly enough to handle processed foods that are available today. Cavemen were genetically accustomed to eating foods readily available to them within their local environments. The physiology and metabolism of modern man has changed very little since the time of our ancestors. Recent changes in our diets due to agricultural advancements have occurred in the last two hundred years. This is not enough time for our genetics to adapt.

Chapter Five: Animals

Hunter-gatherer society focuses on food that was obtained from wild animals and plants as opposed to our modern agricultural society where we rely on domesticated animals. Farmed animals are fed by humans and rely on humans for nutrients for growth and development. Farmers often buy the cheapest products available, which contain processed foods unnatural to the animal's diet. The term "unnatural" refers to foods "not from nature." Unnatural food can simply be processed food like grains or other foods created for animals in order to make physiological changes to fit the market's needs. This could focus on anything from veal, milk, various beef cuts, and chicken breasts to bacon slices. Animals are fed based on what they are being used for. This means the animals are getting their nutrients from foods that normally wouldn't be found if they were on their own in the wild. The animals are fed unnatural substances and develop unnaturally in the process.

Many farmers are using growth products to increase the size of the animal. These products remain in the animal and carry over into what we eat. Men tend focus on red meats as opposed to leaner meats such as chicken, turkey, and fish. Undiagnosed reactions to red meat are common. These reactions can be mild, from gas and stomach pain to diarrhea and malnutrition. Most consumed meats during the Paleolithic era were fish. Gathering was a much more common food source than hunting.

Modern agriculture use is very new in the context of the history of mankind. The change in diet came approximately 10,000 years ago. That amount of time is quite short when compared to 2.6 million years of Paleolithic diet to that point. The hunter-gatherer era was replaced by agriculture. The span of the Paleolithic era is so broad (with movements of people and climate change) that it would be ignorant to think that their diets didn't change throughout the years.

The invention of fire would have revolutionized meals but was thought not to have been used until the last third of the Paleolithic era. Hunting equipment, such as fish hooks, nets, bows, and poisons, were introduced later as well. The general rules of the Paleo diet are the closest match to what is thought to have been the diet of that era. Although the diet may have slightly changed during the Paleolithic era, the general rules still apply, and processed foods were never part of their lives.

Chapter Six: Fruits and Vegetables

The introduction of agriculture affected the way we eat fruits and vegetables. Processed foods are foods that have been chemically processed and made exclusively from refined ingredients and artificial substances. The mass production of fruits and vegetables created problems that could be fixed by using chemical products. An increase in the production of fruits and vegetables has led to an increase in pesticides and fertilizer use. These practices are changing the genetic makeup of the plants. Genetically modified plants are larger, self-pollinating, resistant to insects, and resistant to droughts. Many countries have placed restrictions on the production and importation of genetically modified foods. At this time, the United States does not require a special label to identify a majority of genetically modified foods. Research is showing that many qualities desired using chemicals can be created with safer cross-breeding of wild fruits and vegetables. Certain breeds of fruits and vegetables have a natural resistance to insects. Safe cross-breeding has been performed to successfully create a resistance with some mass-produced crops. Specific breeding can move humans away from harmful chemicals and fertilizers. The Paleo diet excludes processed foods and incorporates natural foods. Foods that are processed include grains, corn, breakfast cereals, cheese, most tinned vegetables, and bread. These foods did not occur naturally in the Paleolithic era. The way grains are processed for consumption could not have been done at that time.

Chapter Seven: The Paleo Diet

The Paleo diet focuses on foods that were available to the ancient people in the Paleolithic era. These foods include lean meats, fruits and vegetables, and nuts and berries. The Paleo diet excludes dairy products, grains, sugars, processed starches, salt, processed foods, and legumes (peanuts and beans). Because the Paleo diet does not include grains, such as wheat, rye, and barley, it's naturally a gluten-free diet. Processed oils, refined sugars, salt, starches, alcohol, and coffee are excluded because they could not be processed during the Paleolithic era. Researchers believe human metabolism has not adapted to the hasty addition of processed foods, causing the increase in diseases we are seeing today. The rules and restrictions for this diet seem complex at first glance. Think about the tools and equipment that were available to the caveman. If a caveman wasn't able to hunt it, catch it, or gather it from the ground, the food is not part of the diet. You cannot hunt or gather a loaf of bread, a glass of milk, table salt, or sugar. You can potentially find eggs, meats, fruits, and vegetables. If what you are buying is in a box, you probably shouldn't eat it.

Chapter Eight: Processed Foods

Processed foods are foods that have been chemically processed and made exclusively from refined ingredients and artificial substances. Processed foods comprise a majority of foods with added ingredients. If the ingredients consist of just one item, it is likely to be a natural food. Processed foods tend to have added sugar, salt, or preservatives in order to increase shelf life and flavor. Bacon is considered a processed food because of the added spices and curing process. A majority of canned vegetables have added salt and or preservatives in order to increase shelf life, which makes it a processed food. Processed foods have added ingredients that aren't natural to the body's digestion. Foods that are microwaveable meals and single-step meals are generally processed foods. If the meal comes in a box, it is a processed food. It is important to stay clear of processed foods because of the chemicals that are added.

Chapter Nine: Foods to Avoid

Dairy

Dairy products are not part of the Paleo diet. A portion of the world is lactose intolerant, and many who aren't still have issues processing dairy. Dairy products can affect our digestive tract, skin conditions, energy levels, allergies, cause heart disease, and can have an impact on hormone levels. Consider that no other species drinks milk beyond infancy. The milk consumed by infants is of nature, often created by the human body. Breast milk isn't processed in any way other than natural body physiology. Dairy products include any kind of cheese, sour cream, yogurt, frozen yogurt, gelato, ice cream, creams, evaporated milk, powdered milk, butter, custard, casein, whey, and milk. Without the intake of dairy, many believe we can't get the nutrients we need. Milk contains proteins, carbohydrates, sugars, vitamins, minerals, and fats. All of these can be found naturally in the fruits, vegetables, and meats within the Paleo diet. Many researchers believe that milk and dairy products should never be consumed. Studies show that up to 75% of the United States' population has adverse effects to dairy products, many without realizing it.

Sugars, Grains

Grain-containing foods are processed foods and generally contain gluten and simple sugars. These types of sugars are simple carbohydrates and should be avoided. The Paleo diet removes almost all sugars from one's diet as well. Not all sugars are bad for you. The sugars accepted are from natural sources such as fruits. Unused sugars are either used in the body quickly as energy or stored as fat. Studies have shown the simple removal of sugars from one's diet can prevent weight gain, control blood sugar, prevent mood disorders, and increase energy levels throughout the day.

Simple carbohydrates are a form of energy that can come from grains such as pasta, bread, rice, cereals. These types of foods could not have been created or consumed during the Paleolithic era. Simple carbohydrates are a form of sugar used in the body and are either burned for energy or stored as fat. They are only stored as fat if they are not used as energy. Simple carbohydrates are fast-acting sugars. If they are not used quickly, they will be stored quickly. These types of sugars do not last as long as the sugars found in fruits and natural foods. So the amount of energy that one gets from simple carbohydrates is short lived, creating quick fatigue after the energy source has been used.

Complex carbohydrates last longer as an energy source and can burn slower in the body, creating a longer, healthier energy source for your body. Simple carbohydrates, such as wheat, rye, and barley, also contain gluten. Gluten is said to negatively affect a large portion of the population with what is being called gluten intolerance. We are seeing an increase in awareness and gluten-free items. Gluten can create medical conditions such as dermatitis, joint pain, reproductive problems, and gastrointestinal issues. As research continues, studies continue to produce evidence that grains can have harmful effects on people without gluten intolerances. Not all carbohydrates are bad. Many carbohydrates that occur naturally from vegetables are appropriate for humans.

Salt

Salt is found naturally in the world; you can find it in oceans and plants, and it is a requirement for sustaining life. So, is salt not allowed in the Paleo diet? Salt is technically allowed in the Paleo diet. The issue is that no added salt is allowed. The majority of salt intake will come naturally from the meats that are consumed. Meats contain larger quantities of salt than plants. The Paleo diet is perfect for getting the required amount of salt for daily intake. Adding salts to meals started with the need to preserve foods and the desire to add flavor to processed foods. Salt is not an unnatural substance, but overuse and excessive use are harmful to the body. Added salt causes fluid-electrolyte imbalances by pulling water to areas of the body where it is not needed or pulling water away from areas where it is needed. Excessive salt intake has been linked to hormone imbalances, thyroid issues, hypertension (high blood pressure), cardiovascular disease, stroke, heart attack, and heart failure.

Starches

The majority of starches are largely found in rice, potatoes, and corn. Although these are vegetables, these foods are farmed and are processed foods. Modern corn is a domesticated vegetable, which means it is man-made and does not grow naturally in the wild. It is thought that corn was domesticated around 2500 BC. Without the cultivation of crops, corn would not be eaten today. Corn is the most commonly grown grain crop in the United States. Potatoes are believed to have been domesticated around 7000 BC. Over the years, farmers have used selective breeding to create over a thousand different types of potatoes. Starches increase blood sugar levels in the human body. As blood sugar increases, our bodies produce insulin to help decrease the effects. Any excess sugar left in the blood stream will be stored in our bodies as fat.

Chapter Ten: Food Recommendations

In most diets, portion control is a necessity. The Paleo diet is one of a few diets that encourages you to eat until you are full and eat as often as you would like. The Paleo diet requires you to eat a variety of foods with a variety of different colors. Different-colored fruits and vegetables contain different kinds of nutrients. When selecting meals, be sure to have a variety of foods from each category of proteins, fats, fruits, and vegetables as well. The Paleo diet does not require a person to count calories. The caloric intake will be generally healthy on the Paleo diet. Removing certain junk and processed foods from your diet can eliminate the need to count calories all together. The Paleo diet will naturally help you lose body fat and build muscle at the same time. This is an all-natural diet, so you will naturally lose weight and show more of your natural body style as you stick with it.

Vegetables

Approximately 50% of your daily food intake should come from vegetables. Vegetables are natural antioxidants and help strengthen your immune system. Eating the recommended daily intake of vegetables can reduce the risk of cardiovascular disease, stroke, and some cancers. Vegetables contain sources of fiber, folate, vitamin C, vitamin K, iron, and calcium. Vegetables act as antioxidants in the body and aid in a healthy digestive system. Vegetables come in a wide variety, which makes meal-plan varieties easier.

Vegetables may be raw, cooked, dried, dehydrated, or fresh. The Paleo diet focuses on groups of dark-green, tan, brown, purple, red, and orange vegetables. The recommended intake of vegetables is 3 cups per day. You can eat as many vegetables as you want.

Green vegetables include the following: asparagus, broccoli, celery, cucumbers, spinach, green peppers, and zucchini.

Green vegetables provide sources of vitamin C, vitamin K, folate, and magnesium. Green vegetables reduce the risk of cancer, lower blood pressure, lower cholesterol, increase immunity levels, and normalize digestion. Red vegetables include beets, red peppers, radishes, red onion, tomatoes, and rhubarb. Red vegetables are an excellent source of folate, flavonoids, and bioflavonoids. Red vegetables are known to reduce blood pressure and cholesterol levels, reduce the risk of cancer, and support tissue growth. Yellow fruits include carrots, squash, yellow tomatoes, and yellow beets. Yellow vegetables are an excellent source of vitamin A and vitamin C. Yellow vegetables reduce the risk of eye diseases, certain cancers, lower cholesterol, lower blood pressure, and promote healthy joints. Tan and brown vegetables include garlic, ginger, cauliflower, onions, and mushrooms. Tan and brown vegetables provide sources of riboflavin, niacin, copper, magnesium, potassium, vitamin D, and vitamin C. Tan and brown vegetables are immune-system boosting and reduce the risk of many cancers. Purple vegetables include purple asparagus, eggplant, black olives, and purple peppers. Purple vegetables are high in folate, vitamin A, vitamin C, and fiber. Purple vegetables support eye health, support digestion, improve vitamin and mineral absorption, fight inflammation, and reduce the risk of cancers.

Meats

Approximately 25% of your daily food intake should contain meats and protein. Proteins are found in all foods made from meat: chicken, beef, seafood, turkey, eggs, and seeds are considered part of the high-protein food group. Grass-fed animals are recommended over grain-fed animals. Grass-fed animals are eating a natural diet. Grain-fed animals have the same problems with wheat as humans. The protein requirements depend on a person's age, sex, and level of physical activity. Most Americans have high-protein diets but are focused on red meats. Protein should come from leaner meats such as fish and chicken. The recommended intake of protein for men is at least six ounces of lean meat per day. On the Paleo diet, you can have more as long as you are getting the recommended minimum.

A four-ounce chicken breast contains the following: 1.4 g of fat, 73 mg of salt, 66 mg of cholesterol, 0 carbohydrates, 26.1 g of protein, 12.4 mg of calcium, and 288.2 mg of potassium.

One can of tuna contains 1.3 g of fat, 46 mg of cholesterol, 521 mg of sodium, 0 carbohydrates, 39.9 g of protein, 16.9 mg of calcium, and 365 mg of potassium.

A four-ounce salmon contains 144 g of fat, 71 mg of cholesterol, 69 mg of sodium, 0 carbohydrates, 25 g of protein, 17 mg of calcium, and 433 mg of potassium.

A four-ounce roasted turkey breast contains 0.8 g of fat, 94 mg of cholesterol, 59 mg of sodium, 0 carbohydrates, 34 g of protein, 14 mg of calcium, and 330 mg of potassium.

A six-ounce beef sirloin steak contains 1.1 g of fat, 11 mg of cholesterol, 12 mg of sodium, 0 carbohydrates, 5.6 g of protein, 3.7 mg of calcium, and 71.9 mg of potassium.

One hard-boiled egg contains 0.9 g of fat, 36 mg of cholesterol, 11 mg of sodium, 0.1 g of carbohydrates, 1.1 g of protein, 4.3 mg of calcium, and 10.7 mg of potassium.

Fruits

Approximately 25% of your daily intake should contain fruits. All fruits that can be found in nature are included in the diet. These fruits may be fresh, frozen, or dried. You can eat fruits whole, cut up, or pureed into a juice or smoothie. The recommended intake of fruits is at least 2 cups per day. On the Paleo diet, you can eat as many servings as you wish as long as you are getting the minimum requirements.

Yellow fruits include yellow apples, cantaloupe, lemons, mangoes, peaches, oranges, pears, and tangerines. Yellow fruits are an excellent source of fiber, vitamin A, vitamin C, and potassium. These fruits reduce blood pressure, lower cholesterol, reduce the risk of certain cancers, support bone growth, and balance acidity in the body. Red fruits include red apples, blood oranges, cherries, cranberries, red grapes, raspberries, watermelon, and pomegranates. Red fruits contain high amounts of fiber, vitamin C, flavonoids, and bioflavonoids. These fruits help lower blood pressure, reduce the risk of cancer, lower cholesterol, and aid in joint support. Tan fruits include bananas, dates, white peaches, and brown pears. Tan fruits contain fiber, vitamin C, vitamin A, potassium, zinc, copper, and magnesium. These fruits reduce the risk of certain cancers, support the balance of hormones, and act as a powerful immune-system booster. Green fruits include avocados, green apples, green grapes, kiwifruit, and limes. Green fruits contain omega acids, fiber, vitamin C, vitamin E, and potassium. These vegetables lower blood pressure, lower cholesterol, reduce the risk of certain cancers, support the immune system, and support vision. Purple fruits include blackberries, blueberries, concord grapes, and plums. Purple fruits contain vitamin C, fiber, flavonoids, beta-glucan, and bioflavonoids. These fruits support the immune system, lower cholesterol, support vision, and fight inflammation.

Chapter Eleven: Oils and Fats

Approximately 10% of your daily food intake should contain fats and oils. Fat and oil intake can come from almost any category of meats, fruits, and vegetables. There is a large myth that fats are bad for you. In reality, fats are essential for heart health and support your overall health. Bad fats, such as trans fats and saturated fats, should be avoided because they raise cholesterol and put you at risk for certain heart diseases. Fats, including monosaturated fats, polysaturated fats, omega 3s, and oils from vegetables, are encouraged and required for body functions. Many people think that oils and fats are bad for you. In reality, fats and oils play a major role in the energy-delivery system. Fats have been made out to be the cause of our own body fat when in reality we are using the same word to describe two different things. A push was made to make foods low in fat, but in order to maintain flavor and shelf life, developers have added preservatives, chemicals, and sugars. Good fats that should be included in your diet come from avocados, olives, almonds, pecans, cashews, soymilk, fish, meats, flaxseed and sunflower seed, and coconuts. Bad fats that should be excluded from your diet come from butter, fried foods, candy, breads, ice cream, premixed products, fast food, snack foods, and baked goods. Fats help store energy, control weight, stabilize mood and brain development, aid in the absorption of vitamins and minerals, and protect our vital organs.

Chapter Twelve: Nutrients

There are many vitamins and minerals needed throughout the body to support and maintain various actions. These nutrients include vitamins A, B, D, E, and K, folic acid, ascorbic acid, magnesium, iron, potassium, flavonoids, beta-glucan, and bioflavonoids. These vital nutrients can be easily obtained through the Paleo diet with the fruits, vegetables, and meats available.

Vitamin B is an antioxidant that supports cell growth, helps the body metabolize proteins, supports the nervous system, and is used for energy. Vitamin B is found in meats, fish, vegetables, and fruits. Vitamin A is needed for vision, healthy skin, bone growth, and the immune system. Vitamin A is found in eggs, green vegetables, orange fruits, and orange vegetables. Vitamin E is an antioxidant that protects body cells and tissues from damage caused by substances caused by free radicals. Vitamin E is found in green vegetables, fruits, eggs, and nuts. Vitamin D is needed for the absorption of calcium. Vitamin D is found in fish, eggs, and the skin when exposed to sunlight. Vitamin K is used for blood clotting and found in green fruits and vegetables. Folic acid is used for making DNA and new cells. Folic acid is found in green vegetables and orange fruits. Vitamin C (ascorbic acid) is an antioxidant that supports metabolism, the immune system, and iron absorption. Ascorbic acid can be found in most fruits and vegetables. Iron helps carry oxygen to all parts of the body. Iron can be found in green vegetables and meats. Magnesium creates energy to help muscles, the heart, and nervous system. Magnesium can be found in most vegetables and fruits. Potassium helps the heart, nervous system, and muscles and creates energy. Potassium can be found in broccoli, spinach, bananas, and oranges. Flavonoids are found in most fruits and vegetables. These are responsible for preventing multiple types of cancers, and they act as a potent antioxidant and as an anti-inflammatory. Flavonoids are found within any fruits and vegetables that have a colored skin. Beta-glucan is found mostly in mushrooms and supports the immune system by encouraging T-cell formation. This helps our body fight against sicknesses and diseases. Beta-glucan is found to reduce the risk of colon and breast cancer. Bioflavonoids are found mostly in citrus fruits and are found to lower cholesterol levels and support joint collagen and fight arthritis.

Chapter Thirteen: Meal Planning

The Paleo diet can be a difficult diet in today's society. It's suggested to ease your way into it while getting rid of the old lifestyle that is still in your cupboards. The pressure and ease of access to eat unhealthy foods is overwhelming. What makes the Paleo diet more difficult is finding foods that are fresh, organic, grass fed, and reasonably priced. Fortunately, there has been an increase in farmers markets and organic brands that are becoming more popular in various areas. Farmers markets can be an option for fresh meats, eggs, fruits, and vegetables that are locally grown and reasonably priced. Spending a little more money for what you're putting in your body can decrease the costs of medical bills later in life. A simple suggestion, when looking for foods within the Paleo diet while grocery shopping, is to stay around the outside of the grocery store. A majority of fresh produce and meats are located around the outside of the store. Getting into the aisles of the store will leave you with processed foods that you want to avoid.

The main food categories of the Paleo diet include meat, fruits, and vegetables. If you are selecting at least one item from each of these three categories for each meal, you will be getting the nutrients you need and following the Paleo diet. You do not necessarily have to select one food for each meal. You may only want to eat fruits and meat for breakfast, have a large vegetable and fruit lunch, and have a dinner with all three categories for dinner. It is important to keep in mind that variety among these foods is important as well. It is not suggested to just eat one type of protein such as chicken. Picking one type of meat will keep you from getting the essential nutrients you need from meats like fish and beef. It is important not to eat only one type or color of fruit or vegetable. Try to get a variety of colors of fruits and vegetables and eat them at different times throughout the day. Every person's body is different, and you many feel differently throughout the day based on the foods you eat at certain times. Be creative with the combinations of meals you can create. A working man can get hungry throughout the day at times other than breakfast, lunch, and dinner. It's important to plan ahead and create Paleo snacks and small meals while you are hungry to get you to the next full meal. Although there is no set schedule with eating, it is often recommended to have breakfast, lunch, dinner, and a snack between each meal. The Paleo diet means eating when you want as much as you want. So if you are hungry, then eat.

For breakfast, is it suggested that you include a fruit, vegetable, and meat. The fruit has natural sugars that will give you the energy boost that you need in the morning. The vegetables are digested more slowly, providing energy and keeping you from getting hungry before your next meal. Meat offers proteins and fats to convert the energy and rebuild or grow muscles. It is suggested to intake more fruits and meats for breakfast than vegetables.

For lunch, a variety of all three categories of fruits, vegetables, and meats can provide you with the nutrients to continue through the day. Fruits will continue to provide the immediate energy needed to get through the work day. Proteins from meats will support muscle use during the day. Vegetables will provide long-lasting energy until the next meal. Eat a variety of colors of fruits and vegetables.

Dinner can be a time to focus less on fruits and more on proteins and vegetables. Fruits can provide too many sugars late in the day. If the sugars are not used, they can be turned into fat for storage. Sugars also provide energy at a time of day when most people are looking for a good night's sleep. Proteins help heal and grow the tissues that were used during the work day. Vegetables provide antioxidants that will help relax the body and calm you before bed.

For the person who is exercising, it is suggested to consume a higher amount food in general to support muscle growth. Eating a small amount of fruits and vegetables can help give you energy during your workout. As you exercise, your muscles are breaking down in order to rebuild themselves. Protein is an important nutrient to add within thirty minutes after your workout in order to provide your body with what it needs.

Following the Paleo diet, you can eat whenever and as much as you want to. Research recommends three meals a day and not eating within an hour of going to bed. Try to break up your meals into three meals a day like normal. If you are feeling hungry in between meals, eat small meals until you aren't hungry anymore as opposed to eating until you are full. This will allow your body to be comfortable while still eating at regular time periods. If your body doesn't eat at the regularly scheduled time, it can become confused, not knowing when or how long it will need to store food for energy. This can create storage or use of energy at inappropriate times of the day.

Chapter Fourteen: Physical Activity

During the Paleolithic era, humans were creatures that appeared to be carved from stone. The men were often very muscular and lean. It is thought their physique was due to long-distance running during their hunts. The American Health Association recommends at least thirty minutes of moderate intensity activity at least five days per week. High-intensity muscle-strength training at least two days per week is also recommended. Exercise plays a major role in any diet when your goal is overall health. The Paleo diet is one component to the healthy lifestyle that Paleolithic humans lived. Frequent exercise and training is the second component that aids in the health advantages of this diet.

Much of the exercise completed during the Paleolithic era was aerobic exercise. Aerobic activity can be described as cardio. Cardio exercise is getting your heart beating faster and your lungs breathing harder. Moderate-intensity cardio exercise could be walking fast, riding a bike, playing tennis, or pushing a lawn mower. Vigorous-intensity cardio activity can include jogging, running, riding a bike, playing basketball, or other intense sports. Muscle-strength training is recommended for men based on their physique goals. Muscle-strengthening exercises include lifting weights, working with resistance bands, and body-weight exercises such as pushups, sit-ups, and yoga. Always consult a physician before starting any type of diet or exercise program.

Chapter Fifteen: Sleep

Getting enough sleep is important for recovering from exercise and rewards you with more energy. Sleep is a form of nutrition for your brain, and your body cannot survive without the mind. A lack of sleep encourages you to make poor decisions with your diet. While feeling tired, you may try to get energy or wake yourself up by grabbing a coffee, energy drink, or eating more than your body needs. Without proper sleep, the human body's metabolism does not work properly. This can cause you to gain weight or store energy at inappropriate times of the day. The lack of sleep creates stress in your body. Stress on your body can cause it to do things it normally wouldn't do. When your body is stressed physically or mentally, it goes into a state of fight or flight. During this mode, your body will gather stored energy in your body for use and slow down the gastrointestinal system. The body does these things in order to prepare for battle. But if your body is in a state of stress from being tired, the body thinks it needs to be ready for battle all day. If the body gets stored energy ready for use and it isn't used, the body will become confused and start to store energy at inappropriate times. The gastrointestinal system is where your body processes and absorbs nutrients. If the body is ready for battle and slows down the gastrointestinal system, the absorption of nutrients will be interrupted, keeping you from getting the nutrients you need.

Chapter Sixteen: Water

Water is important for sustaining life. Water makes up over 60% of the human body. The carrying of nutrients throughout the body would not be possible without water. Human metabolism does not run efficiently without water. Your body has a hard time telling whether it is hungry or thirsty. Many times before bed, people feel hungry. This can be because of dehydration that has occurred throughout the day. People tend to have a late-night snack right before bed, which can actually be harmful to your body. Drinking water can rid you of that hunger before bed.

Conclusion

It can be a challenge to make the drastic change to the Paleo diet. Get a variety of natural foods with various quantities, colors, and flavors. Include at least one food from each category of meats, vegetables, and fruits with each meal. Exclude all processed foods, sugars, added salt, grains, and dairy from your diet. Avoid meats from animals that were fed processed foods. Incorporate exercise into your lifestyle, drink plenty of water, and get the amount of sleep that you need. It's motivating to think about living as our ancestors: hunting, fishing, and living off the land to survive like a real man. These steps will dramatically change your life for the better.

www.ingramcontent.com/pod-product-compliance
Lightning Source LLC
Chambersburg PA
CBHW061944280526
45787CB00004B/1723